Uterine Fibroids:

One Woman's Journey to Healing

Lisa M. Kaminski, MSN, RN

Dedication

This book is dedicated to my mom, Cheryl Weinberger, who has been my strength over the years. She supported me in my fibroid journey as I sought out holistic practitioners and tried new supplements, diets, and therapies for the last 14 years.

To all of my wonderful holistic physicians and teachers, Dr. James Frackelton, Dr. Derrick Lonsdale, Dr. Stan Gardner, Dr. L.B. Grotte, Dr. Allan Warshowsky, Dr. James Silverblatt, and Erin Holston-Singh N.D..

To my patient, caring and understanding gynecologists, Dr. James Guerrieri and Dr. Patrick Quinn.

To my friend Susan Jenovic for listening for 28 years.

To my friend Sandy Brar and her brother for connecting me to the doctor in India and ensuring I received his homeopathic care.

To Chelsea Swick-Higgins for her patience and perseverance in helping with the final editing stages.

Table of Contents

Chapter 1
Me, uterine fibroids and what's available

Frantic internet search, May 2013

Imprisoned on my couch with a heating pad and laptop computer, the search began for options I may not have considered. For many years the pain and heavy menstrual bleeding had been wearing me down. It was mentally and physically draining because I had a life, a family and a nursing career, all of which I wanted to be able to fully participate in.

Being a registered nurse for 19 years served as a good foundation for helping me surf the internet for reputable sites on supplements, physicians, and procedures. Not only a registered nurse, but a holistic nurse by passion. I worked in the conventional confines of the hospital for five years and then I found my calling: nutrition as a means to heal the body. My interest piqued after graduating from nursing school, reading books that enlightened me about a new way of thinking. I discovered things like the fact that eating almonds can strengthen fingernails and that gluten in the diet can wear down the microvilli in the intestinal wall, causing many health issues. (Yes, that was a known fact prior to 1994. . .) But I'm getting ahead of myself—let me backtrack 10 years.

I had taken a low-dose birth control pill to regulate my menstrual cycle for eight years. "The pill" worked pretty well, though I suffered side effects of acne and depression. I cried easily and always felt overwhelmed by life. Then I was hired as a Head Nurse for a phenomenal holistic physician practice in 1999.

Working with amazing holistic doctors taught me many things that nursing school did not. Specifically, I learned that when given the right nutrients, the body can heal itself. This was evidenced daily in the patients we cared for in this very special medical practice. I easily adopted their healthy diet of "God-made" foods. This means fruits, vegetables, lean meats, whole grains and shopping the perimeter of the store; the perimeter has the healthy foods, while processed, boxed, canned, and frozen foods are in the center of most grocery stores.

I started taking some basic nutritional supplements after my visit with one of the doctors. This supplement list included a multi-vitamin, vitamin C, magnesium/potassium, and some minerals that I was found to be deficient in based on a urine test. These supplements, along with drinking plenty of water, daily exercise and 7–8 hours of sleep each night, should have corrected most health issues for me—but my menstrual cycles did not improve.

I read John Lee's book, *What Your Doctor May Not Tell You About Pre-Menopause*, and learned about bio-identical progesterone cream. I asked my doctor to prescribe this wonderful calming cream and it did decrease the bleeding when taken on Days 16–25 of my cycle. . . for a few months. We then increased the dose, and that helped. . . for several months. Eventually I started using the cream daily, which led to some improvement yet again until the severe pain and heavy bleeding returned. Why did the progesterone cream only work for such a short time?

Uterine fibroids, also known as uterine leiomyomas, are benign, smooth muscle tumors of the uterus. They can vary in size and location. Some can cause symptoms for women, yet many women live with fibroids asymptomatically. Symptoms include heavy menstrual bleeding, bleeding between periods, pelvic pressure, constipation, difficulty urinating, pain during sex, miscarriage, and infertility. They usually appear in women between the ages of 30 and 40 years old and are more common in African American women. The cause is thought to be hormonal, such as an imbalance of estrogen and progesterone, or genetic. Fibroids usually shrink once a woman reaches menopause.

Other risk factors include: family history, smoking, nulliparity (never having given birth), hypertension, food additives, soy product consumption, diabetes mellitus, and polycystic ovarian syndrome (Stewart et al., 2017)

Back to my couch in 2013 and my internet search. There is a wealth of products out there, but I needed to know what was legitimate and what was simply advertising. I watched videos and read blogs and testimonials. I found a product called *Neprinol* (a blend of "systemic enzymes") and called the manufacturer, Arthur Andrew Medical, to see what research had been done with fibroids. Unfortunately, there was none, just a few testimonials. The product is touted as being able to break down fibrinogen, which is a component of fibroids, so I kept this in the forefront of my mind and eventually started using it under the direction of a physician. There are several other supplements similar to this.

Medical procedures are not the direction I wanted to take, but if an emergent decision is needed, I must be well-informed and prepared. As a holistic nurse, I am not accepting of what conventional medicine has to offer, except in an emergency. I feel that all of these procedures are too barbaric. Simply removing an organ, while bringing symptom relief, does not cure the underlying health issue that caused the symptoms in the first place. We have to get to the root cause of the problem.

Some women are pleased with the outcome of fibroid surgery and others hold regrets. Some women are happy to be done with bleeding while others are left with lasting complications such as incontinence and sexual dysfunction. All of this should be taken into consideration before making a decision.

I researched endometrial ablation. This is a surgical procedure that involves burning out the uterine lining where the fibroids may be embedded. It is not an option for women who wish to conceive. Many women were fortunate to no longer bleed after this procedure, while others experienced temporary relief, only to need a hysterectomy (surgical removal of the uterus) within five years. This seemed like a possibility to me—if I had to make a quick decision.

Uterine fibroid embolization (UFE) was another procedure I explored. This minimally invasive procedure requires an overnight hospital stay. It involves being injected in the groin with a radioactive dye that allows the physician to view the fibroids. The fibroids are then targeted to cut off the blood supply. It is said to resolve fibroid symptoms in 90% of women; however, its effects on fertility are not clear. There were mixed reviews on this as well. It worked temporarily for some women and not for others. The risks associated with the gadolinium dye meant it was not an option for me.

Hysterectomy is a permanent fix for fibroid symptoms, according to the physicians and radiologist I had spoken to and the research literature. It carries many risks, however, such as infection, hemorrhage, accidental laceration of internal organs like the bowel or bladder, reactions to post-operative narcotics, and more.

There are several types of hysterectomies. Abdominal hysterectomy means that the uterus is removed through an incision made through the abdomen. There is a recovery time of six weeks afterward. Laparoscopic hysterectomy is where the uterus is removed through the vagina. The recovery for this type of surgery is three to four weeks. There is also a laparoscopic robot-assisted hysterectomy, which is considered minimally invasive surgery; recovery time is only two weeks. With any hysterectomy, the physician determines what will be removed. Along with the uterus, the cervix, fallopian tubes, and ovaries may or may not be removed. I would consider this only if I was at the end of my rope. The word hysterectomy terrified me because it is considered major surgery.

Chapter 2
Holistic changes

We have to look at all aspects of our life and see where gradual changes need to be made. Reading as much as possible could help me to accomplish this in my life. Our bodies are burdened with so many chemicals on a daily basis, but we can avoid them if we know what they are. In 2003 I had my five mercury amalgam dental fillings removed and replaced with composite fillings. This brought about immediate relief from my chronic sinusitis: bacteria had been hiding under those fillings, and when we live with harmful bacteria for many years it can lead to chronic inflammation and illness.

Aside from bacteria, mercury has a very long half-life. This means that the vapors from mercury seep out for many years and can cause chronic illness. This harmful effect is heightened when we drink hot beverages, chew gum, or have cracks in the fillings. Think about how close our teeth are to our brain, and imagine the toxic effects.

Mercury filling removal needs to be done by specially trained mercury-free dentists. During this process, chelating pills must be taken by mouth three times per week for several months, to prevent the mercury from reabsorbing into the body. Books on this topic include *It's All in Your Head* by Hal Huggins and *Tooth Truth* by Frank Jerome.

I stopped using fluoride. Fluoride is a known carcinogen, which means cancer-causing. It is present in toothpaste and even in our tap water. We do not need fluoride in our body. Fluoride-free toothpaste is readily available, and both my children and I use it. We have not had any new cavities since switching.

In the kitchen, I initially had a PUR® brand countertop water filter. These filters are changed every few months depending on usage. Eventually, I realized that this filter did not eliminate all chemicals. I then started to get my water from a natural spring in my own glass bottles. The cost may vary at the springs, but ours is only $0.30 per gallon. See www.findaspring.com to locate one near you. I no longer buy bottled water, in an effort to eliminate bisphenol A (BPA) and other toxic plastics from potentially entering my body.

Our tap water not only contains chemicals that we absorb when we drink it but also when we breathe it! Chlorine is harmful to the skin and lungs. By placing a special filter on my shower faucet, it eliminated many contaminants and toxins and I no longer had wheezing whenever I took a shower. I get my filters from Whole Foods Market. They are easy to use and need replacing once per year.

I got rid of as much plastic in our house as possible. This included the vinyl shower curtain: many of them contain volatile organic compounds (VOCs) that tend to give off gas, which we breathe in, for many years. Picture a steamy bathroom and the gases that are expelled from the vinyl shower curtain. There are many shower curtains available now that specifically state "no VOCs," or simply buying a cloth shower curtain is a better option.

Plastic-ware! I switched to glass-lock containers, a much safer alternative to eating foods out of plastic. This is especially important if food is reheated. Once the plastic is heated, it also can become absorbed into the food. Plastic water bottles in our house were replaced by stainless steel or glass with a protective silicone sleeve. The elimination of plastic is probably one of the most important things we can do for our health because once it is in our body, it cannot be removed readily, if at all. Research studies have been done on women with breast cancer. Many of the women were found to have high levels of BPA from plastic in their breast tissue when biopsies were performed. BPA is found in other places, too.

BPA is an endocrine disruptor. It lines canned goods. While I do not use many canned products, I do make my own pasta sauce. I was recently pleased to find that Redpack uses BPA-free cans. I also eat a lot of black olives to get good fats into my diet. I have yet to find them in BPA-free cans or in glass jars. Other olive types, like Kalamata, or green olives, do come in glass jars.

Cash register receipts are especially unsafe to handle due to BPA. In fact, they are purported to be worse than plastic bottles. Blood tests have shown an immediate spike of BPA in the blood after handling these receipts. Here's why: after handling a receipt, if we have lotion or hand sanitizer on our hands, or eat something greasy, the absorption increases. This is according to Mendum et al. (2010), writing in *Green Chemistry Letters and Reviews*. One of the potential ways to remove this from our body is through far-infrared saunas.

Far-infrared saunas can be purchased for the home or found at holistic facilities. They differ from poolside saunas in that far-infrared uses light to produce heat at much lower temperatures than traditional steam saunas. Toxins are then pulled from our body through sweat. The cost to own one is between $1,000 and $1,500.

The microwave! I stopped using one many years ago because of the problems they can create in our body. When we moved a year ago, I decided to leave the microwave in the laundry room, far from where we spend our time for several reasons. The first reason is radiation exposure. Except out of convenience, why would we want to irradiate the food that we eat? The second reason is, studies have been conducted where subjects' white blood cell count (that's an indicator of our immune system function) was tested before and after consumption of "nuked" food. The white blood cell (WBC) count increased after consumption of microwaved food. This is because microwaves use electromagnetic radiation to heat food, and particles tend to move within the food and continue heating it. Our bodies detect that as something foreign and try to fight it off, raising our WBC count.

From the time I got married, I used commercial detergents to wash our clothes. Due to my malfunctioning immune system, I had many allergies. Eventually, I could no longer walk down the soap aisle in the store without sneezing and my eyes watering. This was my immune system fighting these harsh chemicals. Switching to Ecos or Seventh Generation made a big difference in my symptoms and was gentler on my daughters' skin as well.

Endocrine disruptors are chemicals in our everyday life that interfere with and mimic estrogen and testosterone, our reproductive hormones. This can cause early puberty for girls and boys, learning disabilities, reproductive cancers, impaired immune function and more. Over the last 12 years, I have replaced standard personal care products with more natural choices, including hair mousse, shampoo, bath soap, and makeup. I used wonderful smelling shower gels and bubble baths for many years. However, our skin is our largest organ! Whatever we rub onto our skin absorbs into our body. There are no exceptions. This was so hard to give up because I loved all of the great scents. The healthier choices I found include unscented oatmeal bars of soap and shower gels that contain lemon, peppermint, and tea tree oil.

How do you know what's safe to use and what is not safe? The Environmental Working Group (EWG) website (www.ewg.org) is helpful in determining which of your products are safe. You can type in any bath product, cosmetics, nail polish, shampoo and more and it will give you a safety rating. I had been wearing Clinique makeup for 30 years! Since there are no ingredients readily listed on the products, it may not occur to you to examine it. I slowly transformed all of my makeup—except my Covergirl lipstick. I knew I needed to change that too, but it takes time to find the right colors. So I checked my current lipstick on the EWG website and was horrified to find it scored a 9 out of 10 on severe reproductive toxicity! I knew it was not a safe product, but I didn't know how bad it was. What if this was my whole problem? What if it all came down to lipstick? I stopped it immediately and resorted to wearing a natural lip balm for a few weeks.

I chose Mineral Fusion brand for foundation, blush, eyeliner, lipstick, and mascara because it meets the standards for the EWG, i.e. its rating is less than one. This makeup is available in stores and online and costs the same as my previous brand. There are several other natural brands, as well. We have choices! Let's make the best ones in caring for our body.

I hope I haven't lost you yet. This may all sound overwhelming; however, this book is not about a "quick fix." It is about peeling the layers off one at a time and making sure that you are doing everything you can for your body to make it well again. If you truly want to get to the root of your health issue as I did, then please do not give up. You only have one body. . . and this journey applies to all illnesses.

Autoimmune illnesses have risen sharply—by 300%—in the last 50 years, according to Dr. Amy Myers (2015). They are caused by an overactive immune system. Our body fights off things that it feels are invaders. These can be foods, chemicals, clothing, detergents, beauty supplies, and more.

Keep in mind, with each change made, I wait for another menstrual cycle to pass to see if there has been an improvement. This is a very long process since we only have 13 cycles at the most per year. Even if there is no noticeable improvement, know that all the changes are still crucial to improving your overall health. Some changes can take months before improvements are seen.

One of the last changes I made was nail polish. Fortunately, there are some that do not contain the five toxic chemicals, (formaldehyde, camphor, toluene, TPHP, and DBP). Mineral Fusion is the brand I use and is also 100% vegan. I have worn nail polish for 30 years, pretty much nonstop. I recently read how several hours after applying nail polish, a chemical substance appears in the urine. I now felt I had changed everything I could.

Chapter 3
Running out of time: dietary changes and holistic therapies

In July 2013, I experienced my first menstrual hemorrhage, which was terrifying. It lasted eight days and I had to relent and call my gynecologist (he was my sixth). Although I liked him, he did not provide the support I needed. He had his set list of conventional options for me and that was it. I pleaded with him to share anything he knew from his Indian culture, as I was convinced he was holding out on me. I knew if it were his wife, he would find a natural, less barbaric solution than surgery.

He suggested I see one of the "top fibroid doctors in the country," who was local. I agreed and set off to make that appointment. I was not impressed with her, as she did not introduce herself at this first visit. She asked me no questions and proceeded to explain the pathophysiology of fibroids and the options available to me. They were endometrial ablation and uterine fibroid embolization (UFE). She told me we would start with an MRI (magnetic resonance imaging scan) to see where the fibroids were located. I told her I did not want dye used on me for this test. She sighed, commenting that I had my own agenda. Is this a compassionate healthcare professional I want to help me? She said I could have a test performed (creatinine level) to ensure my kidneys could handle the dye. I was more concerned about an allergic reaction, not my kidneys. The visit lasted 10 minutes and I decided this was not for me.

I next experimented with many types of diets to see which would help me. At least twice, I abstained from red meat for six months each time. Red meat, I have been told, can contain red food coloring, an additive, which can cause fibroid growth. This proved to be of no benefit for me, as far as bleeding. Although I ate very little red meat, I switched to a safer, grass-fed beef without the hormones.

I also stopped eating dairy. . . dairy was the love of my life. . . I loved my Jarlsberg cheese every day—that was my lunch. However, I learned that dairy contains a lot of hormones—hormones that I did not need to add to my own excess estrogen.

Sugar causes inflammation in the body, which can irritate tissues and cause fibroids to grow, as well. Sugar also lowers the immune system. I really was not a dessert eater, and sugar was not hard to give up. However, sugar is found in everything. Do you add it to your coffee or tea? If you eat out, fast-food buns contain a lot of sugar. Cereals, dried fruits, baked beans, and so on, contain sugar. Sugar also is disguised under 60 or more different names, such as dextrose, maple sugar, molasses, corn syrup, rice syrup, honey, and fructose, along with many artificial sweeteners. Look them up! If you look at the ingredients of a food product you are eating and you don't recognize the name, you should not be eating it.

Genetically modified organisms (GMOs) are crops that have been altered, specifically corn, sugar, papaya, soy, canola, and zucchini, and are not safe for us to consume. Genetically modified seeds were developed in the 1980s and our foods were forever changed in the

1990s. Seeds can be manipulated to make the crops resistant to bugs, fungal diseases, drought, salinity etc. There are three types of GMO.

The first type is "Roundup® ready" foods, which are bred to be resistant to the herbicide glyphosate. Everything around the plant dies as it is growing, but you end up with a malnourished plant. When we consume these foods it destroys our gut bacteria, which then weakens our immune system. The second type is a BT (*Bacillus thuringiensis*) toxin, a pesticide that is designed to constantly reproduce. The bug eats the plant, its stomach expands and it dies. What do you think happens to us when we consume these foods? Nobody researched this. The third type is a gene promoter. We all have potentially cancerous cells in our body, but this type of pesticide awakens cancer-causing genes. Cancer is said to be the number one killer of children today. So, unless you eat organic produce or it says non-GMO, it is not safe.

Although I did not eat corn itself, it is in everything. My tortilla chips that I love and corn syrup that I'm sure I accidentally eat. Eliminate corn from your diet.

I began to eat a lot more cruciferous vegetables, as in daily. I always ate broccoli a couple of times per week, but now I discovered cauliflower rice. I would run cauliflower through the food processor and then make it into patties with egg and almond flour. This became my breakfast for over a year and then I simplified it by making it into cauliflower rice. This has still been my breakfast for another two years. The value of cruciferous vegetables is that they balance out estrogen in our body. Others include Brussels sprouts, kale, cabbage, collard greens and watercress.

Acupuncture

In April 2013, I found acupuncture. Acupuncture was beneficial to me for several reasons. If I received it when my pain level was high, it would quickly stop my pain, but only for an hour, and then the pain would return. I used this treatment several times a year. Acupuncture was also beneficial because it addressed the issue of liver qi (chi), or blocked energy, which I was told I had. The blocked energy is caused by stress, emotions, or unfulfilled desires in our life. This is an important statement: unfulfilled desires. My marriage had many issues in it for 15–20 years and I was now working in a job that I was not happy with. The doctor told me to leave my husband. That was not possible for me at that time, but I had a feeling deep inside me that he was right, and that unless I addressed that aspect of my life, I would not get better.

The blocked energy contributes to stagnation of your blood. I was advised to use heat packs as needed, eat mushrooms and lima beans, and drink ginger tea to reduce inflammation. A recommendation I did not agree with was the avoidance of all raw foods; I believe we need the enzymes that raw foods have to offer, so this aspect I could not follow. He also recommended a liquid form of iodine. This was extremely helpful to me, as it somehow allowed me to stay up later and not fall asleep while reading to my daughters in the early evening.

Chiropractic

In May 2014, I met with a chiropractor who also specialized in kinesiology. I was in bad shape that day. I had barely made the 30-minute drive to his office and ran to his bathroom only to pass massive clots. This was terrifying to me.

He adjusted my body in areas that he felt needed to be worked on. He also recommended many supplements that I was not already taking along with a detoxification protocol. I felt that the supplements, some of which included cramp bark (*Viburnum opulus*), chasteberry (*Vitex agnus-castus*—which I had a poor experience with in the past), and calcium, made me feel worse.

Calcium is a supplement I do not believe in taking, as I have learned that oral calcium does not go to the bone. Instead, when taken alone, it goes into the bloodstream, which can cause heart problems, and ultimately a heart attack. Research has shown a 24% increased risk of heart attack for women who take calcium pills. It does not apply to dietary sources of calcium. This is according to a paper in the *British Medical Journal* (Bolland et al., 2010) as well as the National Institutes of Health in 2013. However, I recently learned that calcium pills can be taken as long as vitamin K2 is taken at the same time. This is from the book, *Vitamin K2 and the Calcium Paradox: How a Little-Known Vitamin Could Save Your Life*, by Kate Rheaume-Bleue.

The doctor also recommended ice packs for cramping, which did not appeal to me. His rationale was that it helped remove old or stagnant blood from me and allowed the influx of new blood. He told me to eliminate dairy, which I already had, and all sources of corn, which for me meant no more popcorn or my beloved purple corn chips, which I ate daily.

This is also where I met the massage therapist who told me about a book called *The Healing Code*. He revealed that many people he knew had been helped by the book, including his daughter. The "code" involves placing the hands near different areas of the body, which allows energy from our fingertips to heal us. It was implicated in curing people with depression. The author's wife was helped by this technique after medications failed to help her. I found the book at the library and followed the recommendations. It is not a quick fix, but improvements from an emotional or spiritual standpoint can be noticeable after several months. The spiritual component is essential in the healing process.

A few years later I also discovered the emotional freedom technique (EFT), or tapping. This is a type of psychological acupressure that has existed for more than 5,000 years. Tapping on certain areas of your chest and head directs energy into specific meridians while you mentally make positive statements. It is helpful in reducing pain and eliminating negative emotions, among other things.

I also decided to try frequency specific microcurrent (FSM). This is a noninvasive treatment used primarily for muscle and nerve pain. It uses specific frequencies and a micro-ampere current to stop the pain. My pain levels were so high now that I was willing to try this with my holistic doctor, at her urging. I did have some improvement, but it was temporary. It decreased my pain and slowed the bleeding for an hour or so. I tried this twice a week for a few weeks, and then I gave up.

Chapter 4
New doctors and surgery

In July 2014, I experienced my second hemorrhage. It was another frightening experience, which went on for eight days. My gynecologist ordered a complete blood count (CBC) and ferritin (iron) level tests. I was so weak and dizzy, my husband had to drive me. It turned out my hemoglobin was 6 mg/dl and hematocrit was 20 mg/dl. This was very low. The recommendation was that I come in for an iron transfusion if the bleeding did not stop. I actually felt I would prefer a blood transfusion because intravenous iron comes with its own set of risks, such as anaphylaxis. The blood would make me feel better faster. Remember this: it will be important later on.

I waited another day for the doctor's office to call me with a time to go for the iron transfusion. I felt awful at this point. There were moments when I would be back and forth to the bathroom every 5–15 minutes—it was very scary. The bleeding eventually slowed down, but I was so dizzy and my head was pounding. Again, I had to call the doctor back. By this time, the doctor decided I should have a blood transfusion, two units, and stay overnight in the hospital. I saw no reason that I would need to stay overnight, acquire the expense, the risk of infection, and poor quality of care that I have come to know in our hospitals. I told him I wanted it done as an outpatient. He said he would have to check if that was possible. It all worked out without any complications, and I received my two units of blood in the outpatient department. I was still devastated by the thought of having received a blood transfusion because there is the possibility of triggering autoimmune illnesses.

New gynecologist

After this, in August 2014, I felt the push to find a new physician who was more in line with my beliefs. I decided on a very popular, kind physician whom I had heard of for many years. The visit went well—he gave me the same options as the female doctor, but said an MRI was not needed if I chose to undergo endometrial ablation. I kept this in mind and decided to try bio-identical progesterone, 400mg in a pill form. Previously, I had used the progesterone cream, which brought me feelings of calmness.

With the oral progesterone, I did not feel well, as it was a high dose for my petite 100-pound body. I also developed gastroesophageal reflux disease (GERD), or heartburn. It was unbearable. The compounding pharmacist told me it was a possible side effect, as the elevated levels of progesterone cause the esophageal sphincter to relax, which is common in pregnant women. I stopped taking the progesterone.

Planning for surgery

I called my gynecologist and told him I was ready for the endometrial ablation and removal of the fibroids. The bleeding was worsening and I felt confident with him. He was so comforting and assured me it was my decision. Three weeks later, in October 2014, I went in for surgery. He again told me that I could change my mind, but I felt there was no other direction for me to go. He performed an ablation of my uterine lining, but there were no visible fibroids—they were all posterior, i.e., embedded in the uterus. I was disappointed but hopeful that what he did would help me. The pain after surgery was severe and the intravenous fentanyl and oral *Percocet* (oxycodone/acetaminophen) did not relieve it. The nurses were only focused on discharging me, not my pain. I somehow remembered that I had *Midol* (acetaminophen, caffeine and pyrilamine maleate) in my purse. I took two caplets and in 30 minutes I was feeling better and ready to leave.

The book

Recovery was not pleasant, in that mentally I could not shake off the effects of anesthesia for more than a week. However, it was during this time that I remembered the fibroid book I had read a few years earlier, *Healing Fibroids, Naturally*, by Allan Warshowsky M.D, a holistic gynecologist. I grabbed it and started reading my highlighted pages. I felt I now had to go see this doctor wherever he was.

Fortunately, he was only 7.5 hours away in New York. I called his office the next day to schedule an appointment during the Christmas holidays. I was permitted to speak with him for five minutes, as I wanted to know if I could be helped with fibroids that are embedded, or intramural, to which he replied, "Yes."

I continued my search for foods that could help me heal and anything else I may have missed. I was pursuing my Master of Science in Nursing degree and I had access to the online college library. I found that a drug called tranexamic acid was helpful in controlling the bleeding; however, it carries the risk of blood clots. This was eventually prescribed to me. I also found a textbook online about nutrition and fibroids for medical students. That was when I saw the important word that was linked with fibroids: auto-immunity. Women with auto-immunity were more likely to have uterine fibroids. I always felt I may have an autoimmune component, but was never tested for it. This lead me to another search to find foods that would support this.

Spring water and gluten-free diet

Around this time, I watched a week-long series of webinars on the dangers of gluten and its direct effect on many health problems. I adopted a gluten-free diet and began eating cruciferous vegetables daily, limited my sugar intake and drank only water from a deep spring.

Gluten is implicated in so many illnesses. The grains today such as wheat, barley, farro, and millet, are not the same as many years ago. They too have been altered with pesticides to produce a better crop. Put simply, wheat products destroy the microvilli that line the stomach (remember I learned that in 1994?). Without the microvilli, the lining of the stomach becomes leaky, allowing food particles to get into the bloodstream. This is known as leaky gut syndrome. Absorption of nutrients is impaired and the food particles travel to different parts of the body, causing illness. This illness is different for every person—arthritis, migraines, autoimmune disorders, stomach issues—and for me, my uterus.

A word about "gluten-free": this does not mean consuming gluten-free products. These products are even more unhealthy for you than those that do contain gluten (or maybe equally). Gluten-free pasta, cakes, bread, etc. are very high in carbohydrates and contain multiple starches that can create other health issues, like heart disease or high cholesterol.

Off to New York

I arrived in New York in December 2014, eager to know what more I could add to my health routine. It turned out that there was a lot more. I was found to be chronically dehydrated, based on a test performed in their office. I was never a good drinker, although I only drink water.

His protocol included castor oil packs applied to my abdomen, green tea suppositories, probiotics, vitamin B12, curcumin, tinctures, positive thinking, and mindful eating (which means eating without distractions), and more. The rest, I was already doing.

Chapter 5
New plans

I started taking new supplements, including *Myomin* (a Chinese herbal supplement), green tea capsules and suppositories, raspberry leaf, yarrow, and shepherd's purse (*Capsella bursa-pastoris*) drops. I began a 28-day detoxification diet and learned that I felt best eating just vegetables. I became addicted to the protein powder for the cleanse that I was to drink three times per day. It was high in carbohydrates (CHO) and when I ran out, the withdrawal was not pleasant. . . I was irritable and hungry all of the time. I switched to a lower CHO powder until it was discontinued. Then I stopped the cleanse after the 28 days.

A word of caution on protein powders. You need to carefully read all of the ingredients. My recommendation is a physician-grade protein powder, used under the care of a doctor. When using these powders, it is imperative that you drink a lot of water for several reasons. Protein can be hard on the kidneys, and the water helps to flush it out. Also, anyone with a kidney disorder needs physician monitoring as well. Two years after starting on these (I was now only drinking them once daily), I developed kidneys stones. I am the third person I know to develop kidney stones while on protein drinks. I would still recommend them, but with sufficient water intake.

Castor oil packs help to detoxify the liver. I administered castor oil packs 3–4 nights per week. To do this, you need organic castor oil and an organic cotton flannel cloth, both of which are easy to find in health food stores. Keep the cloth folded in fourths and pour about ¼ cup of castor oil onto the cloth—keep it within the center of the cloth so it does not run off the edge. Apply it to your abdomen, near the liver, which is under your ribs on the right side. Cover this with a plastic bag and apply a heating pad. This can be messy! Now relax in bed for at least an hour with your pack. Most of the time, I fell asleep with it on. Then wash the oil off your stomach and store the cloth in a plastic bag. It can be reused for up to three months.

When my lab results came back, they revealed I was pre-diabetic, as evidenced by an elevated hemoglobin A1C (glycation levels over the past three months). Normal is less than 6%. Mine was 5.7%, which is considered high risk for diabetes. This freaked me out, as I was thin and without any genetic predisposition to diabetes in my family. I was told I had to eliminate carbohydrates, or severely reduce them. What?! I loved my carbohydrates. I had already eliminated gluten and dairy, which meant no more pizza or pasta. I had made amends for this, but I depended on beans and rice. . . there was no way I was giving them up. But the fear of diabetes was worse. So, I started to cut back. I am a huge fan of chicken, rice, beans, peppers, onions, and tomatoes; removing the rice and beans, my favorite meal was just not the same.

Why do we crave carbohydrates and grains? Certain foods can create a reaction in the body like the drug morphine. This creates feelings of happiness, sleepiness, and a reduction in pain. These sensations are addictive and make us crave those foods.

According to Nora Gedgaudas, author of *Primal Body, Primal Mind,* "grain consumption causes allergies, food sensitivities, autoimmune disease, celiac, colon cancer, pancreatic disorders, mineral deficiency, epilepsy, cerebellar ataxias, dementia, degenerative brain and central nervous system disorders, peripheral neuropathy, schizophrenia, and autism spectrum disorders" (p. 16). Gedgaudas also explains that our genes do not predispose us to illness, but rather our diet and environment act upon our genes, so we can control 80–97% of our gene expression (our "phenotype").

I also learned that I was autoimmune! I had a positive anti-nuclear antibody (ANA) titer, which indicated the possibility of my developing Sjögren's syndrome in the future. Not the worst of all autoimmune diseases, but I could not believe that this was me. When did things change?

Additionally, I tested positive for two mutations in the gene that encodes for the enzyme methylenetetrahydrofolate reductase (MTHFR). The majority of people carry one copy, but I had two! I had to now research this and found that among many other things, it puts me at an increased risk of developing blood clots. It also means that I have difficulty with detoxification, for example of heavy metals, pollution, and more. Wow—I was not in good shape, from a lab perspective.

I was determined to at least reverse the pre-diabetes and the autoimmunity.

I also learned that my eating should all be restricted to being within a nine to twelve-hour timeframe. Why? It allows the body to rejuvenate itself instead of being in a constant state of digesting.

Think about it—most of us eat pretty much throughout the day, while we work, while we drive, and while we watch television.

This was not going to be fun since I was working on an online Master's degree program and would snack late at night. Not eating was going to be a challenge on those stressful late nights. . . which was every night.

I also realized that I no longer used the treadmill, practiced yoga, or lifted weights. Unfortunately, resuming exercise would have to wait seven more months, until I completed my degree.

Stress was not helping my fibroids. The demands of school, work, and family and the sudden death of our border collie were pushing me over the edge, but I was determined to graduate with honors.

So, I *did* give up the beans and rice, and limited my carbohydrates to no more than 60 gm/day for three months, and then I returned to them in low quantities, like once per week. I was always hungry, and nothing would satisfy me like the comfort of carbohydrates. To give you perspective, a ¼ cup of rice has about 35 grams of carbohydrates and a banana has about 26 grams. That would be all the carbohydrates that I could consume in one day.

It was during this time that Amy Myers M.D released her awesome book, *The Autoimmune Solution*. This was extremely helpful, but it meant more restrictions, like the "nightshade" vegetables and tamari sauce. The nightshades are potatoes, tomatoes, eggplant and some of the starches. These worsen autoimmune conditions, like lupus, rheumatoid arthritis, and myasthenia gravis. What foods am I left with?

Two months later my pre-diabetes had worsened! My hemoglobin A1C was now 6%. But I had effectively somehow reversed my autoimmune status to negative. So I was pleased, but terrified of the diabetes.

My cycles were not what I wanted, but tolerable. The biggest improvement was that I had minimal to no pain each month. This was due to the New York protocol, because after the surgery, I still had a lot of pain for three months.

Water was my biggest downfall. Although my water sourced from a deep spring was very beneficial, I have never been a good drinker. I can go most of the day without a drink because I do not make it a priority. I then found the book, *Water: Your Body's Many Cries for Help*, by Dr. Batmanghelidj. You would be amazed at how many of our modern-day illnesses could be caused by dehydration!

One month before I graduated, my dad passed away suddenly at the age of 71. It was such a shock, as he and my mom had followed the same healthy diet.

I graduated with honors in September, 2015. I then returned to exercise: treadmill, yoga, and free weights.

New recipes

My mom and I searched feverishly for recipes to replace those that we loved. Some included new vegetable recipes, desserts (minimally), and almond flour as a replacement for wheat flour.

Almond flour can be used in cauliflower patties, breaded chicken cutlets, and pie crusts, to name a few. We made our own herbal crackers and later learned how to make nut and seed bars after finding them at a shop in Sanibel.

Some days were good, but other days I missed the foods I had eaten for more than 40 years. It is also time-consuming to make appealing meals while balancing other responsibilities. But our health depends on it and I am committed.

The other factor is that using fresh organic vegetables requires biweekly trips to the store, as we use them quickly and they do not stay fresh for long.

Return to New York, December 2015

My one-year follow-up visit revealed more surprises. My pre-diabetes was gone! Yes, gone—which I can only attribute to my exercise and lower stress levels. I was still eating minimal carbohydrates from time to time. This was great news; however, my autoimmunity was back. This must be the carbohydrates.

New Year 2016

The first five months of this year went well with regard to my menstrual cycle considering I had some major stressors in my life, with a relationship in March, new job in April, and planning a move to a new home in June. This made me think that stress was not a factor. I started eating carbohydrates and nightshades again once per week because I wanted them and I didn't like that I was down to 92 pounds.

Summer 2016

Things did not stay good for very long. By July 2016, I was back to hemorrhaging and in the bathroom every 15 minutes. An ultrasound in August showed no increased growth of the fibroid. Thoughts about this change included the fact that we now lived 0.25 miles from a freeway. Living near heavy traffic can add to our toxic burden of chemicals. Furthermore, my new job was very sedentary, and this can worsen any health issue. Our bodies are meant to be active. Lastly, my marriage had not been in a happy place for a long time. Our bodies can sense this stress, which causes changes in our immune system as well as any organ in our body.

Fall 2016

A call to the New York doctor revealed that all the stress I went through at the beginning of the year had finally caught up with me, and now it would take months to improve. This doctor was against bio-identical progesterone because he said it could make the fibroids grow. I had a hard time with this because I found no research to support it and I liked how it made me feel calm.

By early December, I decided to start on bio-identical progesterone cream again, recommended by my gynecologist and new, local holistic doctor. I felt like I was backed into a corner with no other choices, and my fear of needing a hysterectomy heightened. Unfortunately, the bleeding continued beyond Day 8 while I was using the cream, so I had to stop it. By mid-December, I was ready for surgery. My caring gynecologist only wanted me to choose surgery if I was coming from a position of strength and not weakness. I assumed this was because I would have a better outcome if I was positive. I was falling apart at this time. I was teaching nursing students and would sometimes need to run to the bathroom during class. There had to be something else out there for me.

Homeopathy

In January 2017, my friend Sandy begged me to be treated by her doctor in India. He had helped her sister and many others with endometriosis and uterine fibroids. Money was not important to the doctor—he wanted to help people, as it should be. My friend's brother was the liaison and five weeks later I received *Fraxinus americana* and *Thlaspi bursa pastoris* made by Mother Tincture, along with tiny sugar pills. I was so hopeful and prayerful that these would work. I had improvement in my symptoms within a few weeks: less bleeding but more pain. I tried these for almost three months and then I decided the pain was too much and I would have to stop.

New doctors

In February, I decided to try the bio-identical progesterone cream again. This time I did not experience the prolonged bleeding like in December, and the doctor rationalized that my body needed to adjust. Desperate, in March 2017 I went to another holistic doctor. He recommended iodine capsules, DHA (docosahexaenoic acid, an omega-3 fatty acid), and a few nutritional intravenous infusions. These did not bring about any noticeable improvement.

In April, I found another new holistic doctor. Lab results showed that I had low thyroid activity, or subclinical hypothyroidism. This means my numbers are in the normal range but at the low end. He suggested thyroid medication, sublingual bio-identical progesterone, and low-dose naltrexone to reverse the autoimmunity. He explained that if fibroids are autoimmune, let's reverse the autoimmunity. I opted for all but the thyroid medication. I did not feel I had the symptoms to support it (weight gain, constipation, fatigue, and feeling cold).

By May 2017, I agreed to the thyroid medication Nature-Throid, because the doctor said that sometimes heavy bleeding is caused by a low thyroid and I was willing to try anything. Within a few days, I was no longer constipated, which had been a problem for four years. I started with ¼ grain for two weeks, then increased to ½ grain.

In June, I had a few episodes that I refuse to ever go through again with pain, bleeding and very large blood clots. My gynecologist recommended seeing a radiology interventionist for a uterine fibroid embolization, (UFE). I was tearful at the consultation because every fiber of me was against this, although the procedure sounded promising in that it is non-invasive.

While sedated, a wire is guided through the groin to find the blood supply to the fibroid. This blood supply is then stopped, and the fibroid thus shrinks and dies. What I didn't know is that synthetic balls are injected into each artery to block the blood supply to the fibroid. I could not accept having synthetic objects in my body. Oh, and there is the risk that if they are injected in the wrong place, they could cut off the oxygen supply to your leg, bowel, or ovary. Once the blood supply is cut off to the fibroid, it suffers a "heart attack" due to lack of blood flow and the person experiences 24–48 hours of severe pain. There is an overnight hospital stay. Prognosis varies: some women may do well for several years and others need a repeat procedure.

Naturopath, June 2017

I decided I needed to speed up my path to recovery, yet again. I made an appointment with a reputable naturopath I had heard about for many years. I really liked her and she was very knowledgeable and focused on issues that the other holistic practitioners had not. First, she knew immediately that my liver was where the whole problem started. If we have a sluggish liver, then hormones are going to be affected because the liver manufactures many of our hormones. She also focused on the emotional component and getting in touch with my feelings. She could tell that I was blocking my emotions. This was probably true due to several things that I had been experiencing in my life over the last 15 years. Sometimes you may suppress your feelings in order to function each day with kids and work and life. This is also a much more difficult area to address because it takes time and concentration. I told her that I would have a three-week break from teaching soon and I would focus on my emotions then.

I agreed to the naturopath's protocol, along with stopping the progesterone. I have read conflicting stories as to how progesterone can help shrink or grow a fibroid. After looking at my labs she determined that I did not need thyroid hormone replacement. This was hard for me to accept because although I felt I didn't need it, two holistic doctors felt that I did. She also wanted my iodine stopped because she said iodine can cause cancer. What?

Soon, I realized that after three weeks of thyroid hormone replacement, I had been itching every day, all day. I also felt severe heat intolerance—this could be a symptom of hyperthyroidism. I called the holistic doctor who said to stop the iodine and thyroid medication and then restart the iodine when the itching stopped.

Chapter 6
Issues from birth?

I learned years ago that my mom was given antibiotics for years to treat her acne before she got pregnant with me. Antibiotics cause the loss of good bacteria in the gut. Without those good bacteria, health problems are created. Leaky gut is where it all starts. Without good bacteria and with a lifetime of wheat and grain consumption, the cilia that line our stomach are destroyed. This allows for particles of food that normally stay within the digestive tract to now leak through tiny holes in the stomach. Once this happens, they create problems throughout the body, depending on where our weakest link is. For some, it is digestive issues, for others, allergies, migraines, arthritis, autoimmunity—the list goes on. We are learning now that our stomach has an equal amount to or more neurotransmitters than our brain. Neurotransmitters are involved in major body functions. Think of how important it is to ensure optimal gut health so these neurotransmitters function effectively.

So, if I was born to a mother whose good bacteria were gone due to overuse of antibiotics, then I started out my life without those bacteria as well. This is what contributed to my allergies to pollen and foods from the beginning, and my projectile vomiting as a baby when I was given milk. Doctors did not know what to do about this in the 1970s, so they suggested soy formula, which was not a good replacement (more estrogen).

From the age of 2 to 25, I ate a bowl of cereal on most days for breakfast. Shortly after consumption, I would have a stomach ache.

Imagine, daily, through grade school, middle school, high school, and college. What kind of damage was being done to my stomach and contributing to my allergies and sinus issues?

Not until I gave up dairy and wheat did my gut healing start.

Conflicting opinions

This is a problem when you have too many practitioners working with you. However, as a nurse, I rely on my knowledge and research to make the best decisions for me. Living in Ohio and any of the Great Lakes areas, we are in the "goiter belt." This means that people in this region are more likely to be hypothyroid due to chemicals in the water and a lack of iodine in the soil. Dr. David Brownstein explains this in his book, *Overcoming Thyroid Disorders*. I decided to take the iodine but stop the thyroid medication. It is also important to know what ingredients are in them. For example, Armour® Thyroid, like many medications, contains cornstarch, microcrystalline cellulose and other substances that can cause allergies.

Chapter 7
Prayers

I am a religious person and have prayed a daily rosary for many years. In July 2017, my friend Sue asked me to go to Our Lady of Lourdes shrine, which we are fortunate to live near. She and I were going through similar situations in life then. At the beautiful shrine, we saw testimonials from people who received blessings over the last 50 years. My heart was not in it to be there on that day because I had recently lost a lot of blood and I was weak and short of breath, but I felt at peace.

Procedures

Having another bad cycle in July 2017, which lasted seven days, I decided I needed to prepare for some type of procedure. I planned to follow through with the naturopath because the bottom line is, cutting out a growth or organ may help the symptoms, but it does not help the underlying problem, which appears to be a sluggish liver (according to both the acupuncturist and naturopath), and I needed to get to the root of the problem.

Upon further research for fibroid removal procedures, I discovered focused MRI-guided ultrasound (MRgFUS). Why had I not found this before? I discovered a recent study from November 2016, explaining the benefits which include minimal pain, no overnight hospital stay, and no invasive techniques. This did not seem so bad. I would be on my stomach in an MRI lying on a gel pad. I would receive intravenous fentanyl to manage pain and Versed (midazolam) to relax me. A urinary catheter inserted where they would fill my bladder with water. My rectum would also be injected with ultrasound gel. This is to inflate these organs to better visualize the fibroid. It is an outpatient procedure that takes about four hours. There are basic qualifications that need to be met as well. The prognosis for fibroids appears to be good depending on your age: the closer you are to menopause, the less likely you are to need the procedure repeated. I was 46 years old.

I called the Fibroid Center in Columbus, Ohio for information. The only risk is a potential skin burn that looks like sunburn, and only one patient had that. The downside was that this Fibroid Center just closed due to lack of coverage by insurance companies three days ago! The cost is $22,000. Insurance companies would rather pay for the knife, meaning surgery, than this procedure that has been shown to be effective.

A call to my insurance company resulted in a yes, it is a covered service, the facility is covered as well as the doctor.

There are only a handful of facilities who perform this procedure in the country.

Although the Fibroid Center is closing, the interventional radiologist continued to do the procedure for seven more months in a hospital.

So, I planned to have an ultrasound to measure the fibroid and see if I am a candidate for the uterine fibroid embolization (UFE)—which

I no longer want. After that, it is an MRI with and without contrast dye—which I am totally against, but is necessary.

The ultrasound revealed that I had three fibroids measuring 4.9cm, 4.3cm, and 2.3cm. I met with my holistic physician and told him I stopped the bio-identical progesterone, Nature-Throid, low-dose naltrexone, and iodine. He agreed that if they were not helping that was okay, but the iodine is a must. We both agreed it does not cause cancer. So, I resumed this. He also discouraged me from receiving the dye, but it is required in order to visualize blood flow.

The dye they use is called gadolinium. It is a heavy metal and the side effect is that it can affect kidney function. It has also been shown to cause multiple sclerosis (MS) in people who have received it frequently.

I had the idea to get a prescription for DMSA, or dimercaptosuccinic acid. It chelates metals like mercury, arsenic, lead, aluminum, and also gadolinium. I figured if I took it after the procedure, it would bind to those metals and remove it safely from my body. The down-side is that the capsules are about $8 each and are made at a compounding pharmacy. They can be taken three times per week. A urine mercury and metals test can be taken three months after using DMSA to check the level of metals in the body.

My doctor was kind enough to recommend a free-standing radiology facility. The cost for the MRI would be roughly $900 compared with $2,500 if the MRI was done in a hospital.

The procedure went well. If you have never had one before, you lie on a hard table, then a plate is placed over the abdomen. You are almost completely inside the capsule. It is very cold in the room and the machine is very loud. Lots of clanging and beeping. I received a headset to listen to music. The scan without contrast lasted 20 minutes, followed by another 12 minutes after the contrast was administered. It is important that a pillow is placed under your knees and back, which is the correct procedure. The technician did not give me one under my back and I had pain for several hours afterward.

Consultation in Columbus

The consultation with the interventional radiologist was wonderful. He explained everything in fine detail. We had spoken by phone for an hour earlier in the week. He said I was a candidate based on the type of fibroid as seen on MRI. By this, he explained that mine were dark in color, which meant they were cellular and more likely to be destroyed by the procedure—a good thing.

He only had two concerns about me. The first was that my bowel was blocking the pathway to the fibroid that the laser would be aimed at. The laser cannot go through the bowel or it will damage it. He would not know if the bowel would move out of the way until I was positioned on the table.

The second concern was that since I have not given birth (my children are adopted), the cervix will not dilate enough after the procedure to allow fragments of the fibroids to pass through. This would increase my chance of endometritis or infection after the procedure. The risk for me was 30–50%, which is why it was essential that my local gynecologist was onboard: he would need to be available to order antibiotics should I develop symptoms of infection (cramping, vaginal discharge). If that did not take care of it, I would need a surgical procedure, a hysteroscopy, to remove those fragments.

I was accepting of most of this until I found out that I may not see improvement for two to four months! Nobody I had discussed this with shared this with me. It was disappointing because I was at the end of my rope with these symptoms. I still felt like I needed to have my next plan in place in case the UFE did not work out. That would be a robotic hysterectomy.

Moving on

I did not hear back from Columbus for 12 days, which was not acceptable to me. I pledged I could not go through even one more menstrual cycle. So, I called my gynecologist and told him to proceed with a robotic hysterectomy. His partner was the only one in the practice who performs this surgery. I wanted this because it involved less pain and bleeding and a shorter recovery period. He said he would get me set up to meet with him the next week.

I had to wonder why my journey took me to Columbus for that procedure. I was a candidate, had the right insurance for the procedure, physician, and facility. I have to believe the reason was for me to hear them tell me that robotic surgery was also a good choice.

The history of robotic hysterectomy has some negative points. Sometimes a morcellator was used to cut up pieces of the uterus. In the rare chance that the woman had some cancer cells, they would now be spread everywhere. There were lawsuits about this over the last few years.

A meeting with the new doctor went well. He resembled my dad and even shared his middle name. These were all signs that I was moving in the right direction. I had to have a Pap test and endometrial biopsy done in the office to make sure there were no cancer cells. These came back negative and my surgery was scheduled for four weeks' time. I felt relieved that this would finally be over yet distraught that I would have to go through one more menstrual cycle.

That cycle ended up being the worst in some ways, but each day I found strength knowing that it would be my last and then no more feminine hygiene products ever again. This cycle lasted 15 days. I still need to know why. . . but it wouldn't surprise me if it was caused by stress.

I had also filed for divorce two months earlier. The marriage was not contributing to my health in a positive way. It was not a supportive, loving relationship. I remembered the two doctors who encouraged me to move on from this, and said that I would not get better unless I healed that aspect of my life. They said that I needed to get in touch with my feelings, which I had really placed on the back burner over

the last few years in order to take care of my girls and perform at my
job.

Chapter 8
Strength for surgery

Somehow I found strength from God above and from my dad to be absolutely fearless (well, almost) about this surgery when three months previously I had been distraught. We all reach that point sometimes of. . . enough. For over a year I had said that I could not go on anymore but nobody rescued me from it. I had to make the change; the situation would not change on its own. Between divorce and major surgery, I had felt immobilized.

I placed myself in a mindset where I truly only focused on me and where I was heading with my health. I put my trust in God, my doctors, and the conventional health care that I am not in favor of— and I had a positive outcome. This was only made possible by a book I have now read twice.

A New Earth by Eckart Tolle is one of those books you can read many times and find something new in each time. According to Tolle, "Nonresistance, nonjudgment, and nonattachment are the three aspects of true freedom and enlightened living. Once you see and accept the transience of things, you can enjoy the pleasures of the world while they last without fear of loss or anxiety about the future. When you are detached, you gain a higher vantage point" (p. 225). This was perfect for me because I fight and resist everything. This helped me to sit back and try to let things take their natural course.

I also had to remove my negative thoughts. I was so convinced that surgery would only have negative outcomes and complications, and I had to stop this pattern. I learned that we have an inner purpose and an outer purpose and when we get stressed, our outer purpose has taken over (Tolle, 2005).

This also pertained to my marriage. "As the ego is no longer running your life, the psychological need for security lessens. You are now able to live with uncertainty, even enjoy it. When you become comfortable with uncertainty, infinite possibilities open up in your life. It means fear is no longer a dominant factor in what you do and no longer prevents you from taking action to initiate change. If it is perfectly acceptable, it turns into aliveness, creativity, alertness" (p. 274).

Tolle says that acceptance, enthusiasm or enjoyment must always be present in everything you do. "For now I must accept this, so I do it willingly" (p. 297). And so I accepted that surgery was the right choice for me.

Surgery

The surgery lasted one hour longer than anticipated, I lost more blood than expected and the uterus was "a melon," according to the doctor. But the success was that I was able to have minimally invasive surgery. The pain was very manageable, I had no brain fog afterward, and I had one wonderful nurse and aid in the 24 hours I spent there. I was up walking the next morning. I could not believe it was over. This surgery and recovery was nothing compared with what I had experienced over the last five years.

I did need two iron transfusions and as it was explained to me, blood is used as a last resort due to the risk of infections. I had previously read that iron caused anaphylactic reactions, but now they use iron sucrose and that is not the case. If only my previous doctor had taken the time to explain that to me when I ended up with a blood transfusion in 2014.

Fast forward three months after surgery. Upon awakening each morning, I drink a glass of spring water with lemon, pray, do 10 minutes of yoga, then 20 minutes on the treadmill and I feel great to start my day.

I feel I had a quick recovery because of the processed food, chemicals, dairy, and gluten I had eliminated from my diet. So all that I did these past few years was not unnecessary.

Tips after surgery

As a nurse, I feel it is important to share with you how to have the best recovery:

- Find someone to stay with you in the hospital, to be your spokesperson.

- Drink plenty of water (at least half your weight in ounces per day, e.g., if you   weigh 100lbs, drink 50oz of water every day).

- Use your incentive spirometer, a device to prevent pneumonia, every hour.

- Take the pain medication offered to you.

- Get up and walk as soon as allowed to prevent a blood clot.

- Chew gum if you have shoulder pain; this is caused by the gas the surgeon instilled in you during surgery.

- When you get home, walk around every few hours.

- Eat foods high in fiber (fruits, vegetables, whole wheat bread, oatmeal etc.); the pain medication they give you slows bowel activity down. If you get to the fourth day without a bowel movement, take action: can you switch from a narcotic (opioid) to ibuprofen? Keep moving and drink plenty of water.

Healing the liver

When I agreed to the surgery, I knew that it would not be the end of everything. The only thing that happened was my uterus was removed, and that was what had been causing my symptoms. Yes, I am thrilled to not experience those symptoms anymore. However, it will be up to me and my holistic doctors to resolve the rest of this. I still need to maintain the grain-free, dairy-free, low-carbohydrate diet.

Remember, I have a sluggish liver, or liver qi (chi), depending on which practitioner I speak to. This pertains to anyone who has hormonal issues. There are many ways to fix this. Acupuncture is very effective, castor oil packs to the abdomen, and supplements that support the liver, such as diindolylmethane (DIM), an antioxidant and phytonutrient that is found in cruciferous vegetables.

I also have two copies of the MTHFR gene, which means I have difficulty detoxifying, so it will take time to detoxify.

The final piece

But first, I need the finality of becoming whole again from my marriage. I cannot stress this point enough in the healing process. Whether it is unhappiness, abuse, unhealthy relationships, anger, work issues, whatever—nothing will change unless these things are removed from your life. Being in a loving, supportive relationship is key to making improvements in your health. I truly believe that all of the protocols I used would have had a heightened effect if my stressors could have been diminished or eliminated. It doesn't matter if you take a lot of supplements and eat a pure diet. Our brain knows when things are not right and our mind-body connection is very strong.

Overall, I feel that the majority of the therapies I tried benefitted me in some way. I would use all of them again if I had the choice, except for one: I would omit the bio-identical progesterone cream. Doctors are divided over whether it is beneficial or harmful. I had a mixed experience with it: in the early years I felt very calm from it, and it lessened my bleeding—yet in later years, I feel it increased the bleeding. I would also recommend the avoidance of tampons, as they can cause stagnation of the blood and thus potentially increase the risk of developing fibroids.

You will have to decide what is best for you. My belief is to keep it holistic as much as possible and for as long as you can tolerate the symptoms. If things are not moving in a positive direction, a robotic hysterectomy, if you are a candidate, is not a bad way to go. I would have chosen this several years earlier had I known how easy the recovery would be for me.

You

Depending on where you are on this whole spectrum, there are so many things to keep in mind.

First, not everyone will end up having a hysterectomy like I did. If I had handled my marriage differently, I truly believe I could have healed this without surgery. My first goal in writing this book is my hope that you can be healed without these procedures.

For some, nutrition, supplements, and exercise alone may work.

For others, like my mom who had fibroids, a birth control pill may work.

However, for everyone, nutrition and the elimination of toxins from everyday life foods and household products is crucial to getting to the root of this. This is your starting point.

My second goal in writing this book is to show you what is available, how to get to the root cause of uterine fibroids and to save you time. Hopefully, my book will bring you to your resolution faster than the 14 years it took me.

Chapter 9
Summary of holistic therapies and treatments

- **Diet – clean it up**

    o no processed foods or fast foods

    o no dairy, grains (wheat, barley, millet, rice, etc), sugar, or corn products

    o possibly no to low carbohydrates or nightshade vegetables

    o eat fresh organic fruits and vegetables, especially cruciferous (broccoli, cauliflower, Brussels sprouts)

    o lean grass-fed meats and wild fish

    o lots of pure spring water

- **Supplements – see next section for my recommendations**

- **Acupuncture**

- **Energy medicine** (reiki, jin shin jyutsu, frequency microcurrent stimulation (FSM))

- **Detoxify**

    o Use elimination diets

    o Castor oil packs

- **Eliminate heavy metals**

    o Safely have mercury amalgam dental fillings removed

    o Detoxify heavy metals with oral or intravenous chelators

- **Eliminate endocrine disruptors and other chemicals**

- o Electromagnetic fields (EMFs)
- o Microwaves, cell phones in close contact with your body, computers
- o Fluoride
- o Use shower faucet filters
- o No plastics/BPA
- o Hair, bath, and body products, detergents, makeup, nail polish

- **Spiritual**
  - o Get rid of anything in your life that you cannot accept, feel joy or enthusiasm about. This is the most important thing you can do for yourself.
  - o Practice nonresistance, nonjudgment, and non-attachment
  - o Prayer
  - o Meditation
  - o Yoga
  - o "The healing code"
  - o Emotional freedom technique – tapping

- **Lab work**
  - o CBC
  - o BMP
  - o Vitamin D3 level (optimize at 80mg/dl)
  - o Vitamin B12 level
  - o Autoimmune (ANA titer, RF, ESR)

- o   Thyroid (TSH, T3, T4, reverse T3)

- o   Methylation mutation

- o   Urine mercury and metals test

- **Conventional medical treatments – if nothing else has worked**

  - o   Endometrial ablation

  - o   Uterine fibroid embolization (UFE)

  - o   MRI-guided focused ultrasound (MRgFUS)

  - o   Robotic hysterectomy

Nutritional supplement recommendations

NB. All of these should be used under the guidance of a holistic physician after lab testing has been done. They should all be free of gluten, dairy, soy, corn, wheat, yeast, artificial colors, flavors or fillers.

- High quality multi-vitamin

- Probiotics 50 billion units

- Vitamin D3 5,000 units

- Vitamin K2 90mcg (helps absorb the D3)

- Vitamin C 2,000-3,000mg/day

- Vitamin B complex

- Vitamin B12 5,000mcg (methylcobalamin)

- Curcumin 1,000mg or higher

- Magnesium/potassium complex

- Iodine

* Zinc 50mg

* Selenium 200mcg

References and recommended reading

Batmanghelidj, W. (2008). *Your Body's Many Cries for Water*. 3rd edn. Falls Church, VA: Global Health Solutions.

Bolland, M.J., Avenell, A., Baron, J.A., Grey, A., MacLennan, G.S., Gamble, G.D. and Reid, I.R. (2010). 'Effect of calcium supplements on risk of myocardial infarction and cardiovascular events: meta-analysis', *British Medical Journal*, 341: c3691. doi: https://doi.org/10.1136/bmj.c3691.

Brogan, K. (2016). *A Mind of Your Own: The Truth About Depression and How Women Can Heal Their Bodies to Reclaim Their Lives*. New York: Harper Wave.

Brownstein, D. (2002). *Overcoming Thyroid Disorders*. 2nd edn. West Bloomfield, MI: Medical Alternatives Press, Inc.

Environmental Health Perspectives. (2012). *Bisphenol A*. Available at: https://ehp.niehs.nih.gov/wp-content/uploads/2012/10/EHP-Collection-Bisphenol-A.pdf

Environmental Working Group home page: https://www.ewg.org

Fife, B. (2004). *The Coconut Oil Miracle*. Colorado Springs: Piccadilly Books.

Find a Spring home page: www.findaspring.com/

Gedgauda, N. (2011). *Primal Body, Primal Mind: Beyond the Paleo Diet for Total Health and a Longer Life*. Rochester, VT: Healing Arts Press.

Huggins, H.A. (1993). *It's All in Your Head: The Link Between Mercury Amalgams and Illness*. New York: Avery.

Jerome, F. (1996). *Tooth Truth: A Patient's Guide to Metal-free Dentistry*. San Diego: ProMotion Publishing.

Lee, J. (1999). *What Your Doctor May Not Tell You About Pre-Menopause: Balance Your Hormones and Your Life From Thirty to Fifty*. New York: Warner Books.

Loyd, A. and Johnson, B. (2012). *The Healing Code*. Peoria, AZ: Intermedia Publishing Group.

Mendum, T., Stoler, E., VanBenschoten, H. and Warner, J.C. (2010). 'Concentration of bisphenol A in thermal paper', *Green Chemistry Letters and Reviews*, 4(1): 81–86. doi: 10.1080/17518253.2010.502908

Myers, A. (2015). *The Autoimmune Solution: Prevent and Reverse the Full Spectrum of Inflammatory Symptoms and Diseases*. New York: Harper Collins.

Newport, M. (2011). *Alzheimer's Disease: What if There Was a Cure? The Story of Ketones*. Laguna Beach, CA: Basic Health Publications, Inc.

Perlmutter, D. and Loberg, K. (2013). *Grain Brain: The Surprising Truth about Wheat, Carbs, and Sugar—Your Brain's Silent Killers*. New York: Little, Brown and Company.

Radiology Society of North America. Information resource for patients: https://www.radiologyinfo.org

Rheaume-Bleue, K. (2013). *Vitamin K2 and the Calcium Paradox: How a Little-Known Vitamin Could Save Your Life*. Mississauga, Ont.: John Wiley & Sons Canada

Somers, S. (2016). TOX-SICK: From Toxic to Not Sick. New York: Harmony Books.

Stewart, E.A., Cookson, C.L., Gandolfo, R.A. and Schulze-Rath, R. (2017). 'Epidemiology of Uterine Fibroids: A Systemic Review', *BJOG: An International Journal of Obstetrics and Gynaecology*, 124(10): 1501–1512. doi 10.1111/1471-0528.14640

Tolle, E. (2005). A New Earth. London: Penguin Books.

Warshowsky, A. and Oumano, E. (2002). Healing Fibroids: A Doctor's Guide to a Natural Cure. New York: Fireside.

About the author

Lisa M. Kaminski has been a registered nurse for 25 years. She has a passion for nutrition and holistic-based therapies and believes that the body can heal itself when given the right nutrients and spiritual care. She has worked with several holistic physicians for 18 years.

She has a Master of Science in Nursing, with a focus on education. She received certifications over the years in chelation therapy and hyperbaric oxygen therapy and is a holistic health advisor and corporate wellness coach. She is currently pursuing a certificate for Adult Gerontology Nurse Practitioner.

Her desire is to help individuals and corporations achieve wellness and to ultimately reduce our current drain on medical health spending. Her goal is to help prevent illness by empowering others to be proactive with diet, exercise, and lifestyle choices.

She currently works as nursing faculty at a local college and with holistic physicians. In her free time, she enjoys ballroom dancing, especially Argentine Tango. She resides in Cleveland, Ohio with her two daughters and two cats.